CW00385986

PERSONAL DET(

Name: ....

Birthday: ....

Allergies: ....

Blood Type: ....

Weight: ....

Height: ....

Diagnoses: ....

Contact Number: ....

Address: ....

Additional Info: ....

Emergency Contact

Name: ....

Phone: ....

Relationship: ....

Details: ....

NOTES

NOTES

DATE: ....

CHEMO DRUG: ....

DAY # ....   AFTER CHEMO # ....

TODAY I FEEL

....

....

....

....

EXERCISE
☐
☐
☐

FOOD & DRINK
☐
☐
☐

SLEEP
☐
☐
☐

GRATITUDE

NOTES

....

....

....

....

....

....

TIME	MEDICATION	DOSAGE	REACTIONS

DATE: ....

CHEMO DRUG: ....

DAY # .... AFTER CHEMO # ....

TODAY I FEEL

....

....

....

....

EXERCISE ☐ ☐ ☐

FOOD & DRINK ☐ ☐ ☐

SLEE ☐ ☐ ☐

GRATITUDE

NOTES

TIME	MEDICATION	DOSAGE	REACTIONS

DATE: ....

CHEMO DRUG: ....

DAY # ....   AFTER CHEMO # ....

TODAY I FEEL

....
....
....
....
....

EXERCISE
- [ ]
- [ ]
- [ ]

FOOD & DRINK
- [ ]
- [ ]
- [ ]

SLE
- [ ]
- [ ]

GRATITUDE

NOTES

....
....
....
....
....
....
....

TIME	MEDICATION	DOSAGE	REACTIONS

DATE: ....

CHEMO DRUG: ....

DAY # ....   AFTER CHEMO # ....

TODAY I FEEL

....

....

....

....

EXERCISE

☐
☐
☐

FOOD & DRINK

☐
☐
☐

SLEEP

☐
☐
☐

GRATITUDE

NOTES

....

....

....

....

....

....

....

TIME	MEDICATION	DOSAGE	REACTIONS

DATE: ....

CHEMO DRUG: ....

DAY # ....   AFTER CHEMO # ....

TODAY I FEEL

....

....

....

....

EXERCISE   FOOD & DRINK   SLEEP

☐   ☐   ☐

☐   ☐   ☐

☐   ☐   ☐

GRATITUDE   ☐ ☐ ☐ ☐ ☐ ☐

NOTES

....

....

....

....

....

....

TIME	MEDICATION	DOSAGE	REACTIONS

DATE: ....

CHEMO DRUG: ....

DAY # .... AFTER CHEMO # ....

TODAY I FEEL

....

....

....

....

EXERCISE

☐
☐
☐

FOOD & DRINK

☐
☐
☐

SLEE

☐
☐
☐

GRATITUDE

NOTES

....

....

....

....

....

....

TIME	MEDICATION	DOSAGE	REACTIONS

DATE: ....

CHEMO DRUG: ....

DAY # .... AFTER CHEMO # ....

TODAY I FEEL

....

....

....

....

EXERCISE

☐
☐
☐

FOOD & DRINK

☐
☐
☐

SLEEP

☐
☐
☐

GRATITUDE

NOTES

....

....

....

....

....

....

....

TIME	MEDICATION	DOSAGE	REACTIONS

DATE: ....

CHEMO DRUG: ....

DAY # ....　　　　AFTER CHEMO # ....

TODAY I FEEL

....

....

....

....

EXERCISE
☐
☐
☐

FOOD & DRINK
☐
☐
☐

SLEEP
☐
☐
☐

GRATITUDE

NOTES

....

....

....

....

....

....

TIME	MEDICATION	DOSAGE	REACTIONS

DATE: ....

CHEMO DRUG: ....

DAY # ....   AFTER CHEMO # ....

TODAY I FEEL

....

....

....

....

EXERCISE   FOOD & DRINK   SLEE

☐   ☐   ☐
☐   ☐   ☐
☐   ☐   ☐

GRATITUDE

NOTES

....

....

....

....

....

....

TIME	MEDICATION	DOSAGE	REACTIONS

DATE: ....

CHEMO DRUG: ....

DAY # .... AFTER CHEMO # ....

TODAY I FEEL

....
....
....
....

EXERCISE
☐
☐
☐

FOOD & DRINK
☐
☐
☐

SLEE
☐
☐
☐

GRATITUDE

NOTES

TIME	MEDICATION	DOSAGE	REACTIONS

DATE: ....

CHEMO DRUG: ....

DAY # ....   AFTER CHEMO # ....

TODAY I FEEL

....

....

....

....

EXERCISE
- [ ]
- [ ]
- [ ]

FOOD & DRINK
- [ ]
- [ ]
- [ ]

SLE[
- [ ]
- [ ]
- [ ]

GRATITUDE

NOTES

....

....

....

....

....

....

....

TIME	MEDICATION	DOSAGE	REACTIONS

DATE: ....

CHEMO DRUG: ....

DAY # .... AFTER CHEMO # ....

TODAY I FEEL

....
....
....
....

EXERCISE
- [ ]
- [ ]
- [ ]

FOOD & DRINK
- [ ]
- [ ]
- [ ]

SLEEP
- [ ]
- [ ]
- [ ]

GRATITUDE

NOTES

....
....
....
....
....
....

TIME	MEDICATION	DOSAGE	REACTIONS

DATE: _____

CHEMO DRUG: _____

DAY # _____   AFTER CHEMO # _____

TODAY I FEEL

_____
_____
_____
_____

EXERCISE   FOOD & DRINK   SLEE
☐   ☐   ☐
☐   ☐   ☐
☐   ☐   ☐

GRATITUDE

NOTES

_____
_____
_____
_____
_____
_____
_____

TIME	MEDICATION	DOSAGE	REACTIONS

DATE: ....

CHEMO DRUG: ....

DAY # ....   AFTER CHEMO # ....

TODAY I FEEL

EXERCISE

☐
☐
☐

FOOD & DRINK

☐
☐
☐

SLEE

☐
☐
☐

GRATITUDE

NOTES

TIME	MEDICATION	DOSAGE	REACTIONS

DATE: ....

CHEMO DRUG: ....

DAY # ....   AFTER CHEMO # ....

TODAY I FEEL

....

....

....

....

EXERCISE   FOOD & DRINK   SLEEP

☐   ☐   ☐

☐   ☐   ☐

☐   ☐   ☐

GRATITUDE

NOTES

....

....

....

....

....

....

TIME	MEDICATION	DOSAGE	REACTIONS

DATE: ....

CHEMO DRUG: ....

DAY # ....   AFTER CHEMO # ....

TODAY I FEEL

....

....

....

....

EXERCISE

☐
☐
☐

FOOD & DRINK

☐
☐
☐

SLEE

☐
☐
☐

GRATITUDE

NOTES

....

....

....

....

....

....

TIME	MEDICATION	DOSAGE	REACTIONS

DATE: ....

CHEMO DRUG: ....

DAY # ....   AFTER CHEMO # ....

TODAY I FEEL

....
....
....
....

EXERCISE
- [ ]
- [ ]
- [ ]

FOOD & DRINK
- [ ]
- [ ]
- [ ]

SLE[
- [ ]
- [ ]
- [ ]

GRATITUDE

NOTES

TIME	MEDICATION	DOSAGE	REACTIONS

DATE: ....

CHEMO DRUG: ....

DAY # ....   AFTER CHEMO # ....

TODAY I FEEL

....

....

....

....

EXERCISE
- [ ]
- [ ]
- [ ]

FOOD & DRINK
- [ ]
- [ ]
- [ ]

SLEEP
- [ ]
- [ ]
- [ ]

GRATITUDE

NOTES

....

....

....

....

....

TIME	MEDICATION	DOSAGE	REACTIONS

DATE: ....

CHEMO DRUG: ....

DAY # ....   AFTER CHEMO # ....

TODAY I FEEL

EXERCISE   FOOD & DRINK   SLEE

☐   ☐   ☐

☐   ☐   ☐

☐   ☐   ☐

GRATITUDE

NOTES

TIME	MEDICATION	DOSAGE	REACTIONS

DATE: ....

CHEMO DRUG: ....

DAY # ....   AFTER CHEMO # ....

TODAY I FEEL

EXERCISE

☐
☐
☐

FOOD & DRINK

☐
☐
☐

SLEE

☐
☐

GRATITUDE

NOTES

TIME	MEDICATION	DOSAGE	REACTIONS

DATE: ....

CHEMO DRUG: ....

DAY # ....   AFTER CHEMO # ....

TODAY I FEEL

_____

_____

_____

_____

EXERCISE   FOOD & DRINK   SLEEP

☐   ☐   ☐

☐   ☐   ☐

☐   ☐   ☐

GRATITUDE

NOTES

_____

_____

_____

_____

_____

_____

TIME	MEDICATION	DOSAGE	REACTIONS

DATE: ....

CHEMO DRUG: ....

DAY # ....   AFTER CHEMO # ....

TODAY I FEEL

....

....

....

....

EXERCISE   FOOD & DRINK   SLEE

☐   ☐   ☐
☐   ☐   ☐
☐   ☐   ☐

GRATITUDE

NOTES

....

....

....

....

....

....

....

....

TIME	MEDICATION	DOSAGE	REACTIONS

DATE: _____

CHEMO DRUG: _____

DAY # _____ AFTER CHEMO # _____

TODAY I FEEL

_____
_____
_____
_____

EXERCISE

☐
☐
☐

FOOD & DRINK

☐
☐
☐

SLEE

☐
☐
☐

GRATITUDE

NOTES

_____
_____
_____
_____
_____
_____
_____

TIME	MEDICATION	DOSAGE	REACTIONS

DATE: ....

CHEMO DRUG: ....

DAY # .... AFTER CHEMO # ....

TODAY I FEEL

EXERCISE
☐
☐
☐

FOOD & DRINK
☐
☐
☐

SLEE
☐
☐
☐

GRATITUDE

NOTES

TIME	MEDICATION	DOSAGE	REACTIONS

DATE: ....

CHEMO DRUG: ....

DAY # ....   AFTER CHEMO # ....

TODAY I FEEL

....

....

....

....

EXERCISE
☐
☐
☐

FOOD & DRINK
☐
☐
☐

SLEE
☐
☐
☐

GRATITUDE

NOTES

....

....

....

....

....

....

....

....

....

TIME	MEDICATION	DOSAGE	REACTIONS

DATE: ....

CHEMO DRUG: ....

DAY # ....   AFTER CHEMO # ....

TODAY I FEEL

....

....

....

....

EXERCISE   FOOD & DRINK   SLE

☐   ☐   ☐

☐   ☐   ☐

☐   ☐   ☐

GRATITUDE

NOTES

TIME	MEDICATION	DOSAGE	REACTIONS

DATE: ....

CHEMO DRUG: ....

DAY # ....   AFTER CHEMO # ....

TODAY I FEEL

....

....

....

....

EXERCISE   FOOD & DRINK   SLEEP

☐   ☐   ☐
☐   ☐   ☐
☐   ☐   ☐

GRATITUDE

NOTES

....

....

....

....

....

....

....

TIME	MEDICATION	DOSAGE	REACTIONS

DATE: ....

CHEMO DRUG: ....

DAY # ....   AFTER CHEMO # ....

TODAY I FEEL

....

....

....

....

EXERCISE   FOOD & DRINK   SLEE

☐   ☐   ☐
☐   ☐   ☐
☐   ☐   ☐

GRATITUDE

NOTES

....

....

....

....

....

....

....

TIME	MEDICATION	DOSAGE	REACTIONS

DATE: ....

CHEMO DRUG: ....

DAY # ....   AFTER CHEMO # ....

TODAY I FEEL

....

....

....

....

EXERCISE
- [ ]
- [ ]
- [ ]

FOOD & DRINK
- [ ]
- [ ]
- [ ]

SLE[
- [ ]
- [ ]
- [ ]

GRATITUDE

NOTES

....

....

....

....

....

TIME	MEDICATION	DOSAGE	REACTIONS

DATE: ....

CHEMO DRUG: ....

DAY # ....   AFTER CHEMO # ....

TODAY I FEEL

....

....

....

....

EXERCISE   FOOD & DRINK   SLEEF

☐   ☐   ☐

☐   ☐   ☐

☐   ☐   ☐

GRATITUDE

◇ ◇ ◇ ◇ ◇ ◇

NOTES

....

....

....

....

....

....

TIME	MEDICATION	DOSAGE	REACTIONS

DATE: ....

CHEMO DRUG: ....

DAY # ....   AFTER CHEMO # ....

TODAY I FEEL

EXERCISE
☐
☐
☐

FOOD & DRINK
☐
☐
☐

SLEE
☐
☐
☐

GRATITUDE

NOTES

TIME	MEDICATION	DOSAGE	REACTIONS

DATE: ....

CHEMO DRUG: ....

DAY # ....   AFTER CHEMO # ....

TODAY I FEEL

....

....

....

....

EXERCISE
- [ ]
- [ ]
- [ ]

FOOD & DRINK
- [ ]
- [ ]
- [ ]

SLEE
- [ ]
- [ ]
- [ ]

GRATITUDE

NOTES

....

....

....

....

....

....

TIME	MEDICATION	DOSAGE	REACTIONS

DATE: ....

CHEMO DRUG: ....

DAY # ....   AFTER CHEMO # ....

TODAY I FEEL

....
....
....
....

EXERCISE   FOOD & DRINK   SLEEP

☐   ☐   ☐
☐   ☐   ☐
☐   ☐   ☐

GRATITUDE

NOTES

....
....
....
....
....
....

TIME	MEDICATION	DOSAGE	REACTIONS

DATE: ....

CHEMO DRUG: ....

DAY # .... AFTER CHEMO # ....

TODAY I FEEL

....

....

....

....

EXERCISE   FOOD & DRINK   SLEE

☐   ☐   ☐
☐   ☐   ☐
☐   ☐   ☐

GRATITUDE

NOTES

....

....

....

....

....

....

....

TIME	MEDICATION	DOSAGE	REACTIONS

DATE: ....

CHEMO DRUG: ....

DAY # ....　　　AFTER CHEMO # ....

TODAY I FEEL

EXERCISE
- [ ]
- [ ]
- [ ]

FOOD & DRINK
- [ ]
- [ ]
- [ ]

SLE[
- [ ]
- [ ]

GRATITUDE

NOTES

TIME	MEDICATION	DOSAGE	REACTIONS

DATE: ....

CHEMO DRUG: ....

DAY # .... AFTER CHEMO # ....

TODAY I FEEL

....

....

....

....

EXERCISE   FOOD & DRINK   SLEE

☐   ☐   ☐
☐   ☐   ☐
☐   ☐   ☐

GRATITUDE

NOTES

....

....

....

....

....

....

....

....

TIME	MEDICATION	DOSAGE	REACTIONS

DATE: ....

CHEMO DRUG: ....

DAY # .... AFTER CHEMO # ....

TODAY I FEEL

....

....

....

....

EXERCISE
- [ ]
- [ ]
- [ ]

FOOD & DRINK
- [ ]
- [ ]
- [ ]

SLEE
- [ ]
- [ ]
- [ ]

GRATITUDE

NOTES

....

....

....

....

....

....

....

....

TIME	MEDICATION	DOSAGE	REACTIONS

DATE: ....

CHEMO DRUG: ....

DAY # ....   AFTER CHEMO # ....

TODAY I FEEL

....
....
....
....

EXERCISE
☐
☐
☐

FOOD & DRINK
☐
☐
☐

SLE[
☐
☐
☐

GRATITUDE

NOTES

....
....
....
....
....
....
....

TIME	MEDICATION	DOSAGE	REACTIONS

DATE: ....

CHEMO DRUG: ....

DAY # .... AFTER CHEMO # ....

TODAY I FEEL

....
....
....
....

EXERCISE

☐
☐
☐

FOOD & DRINK

☐
☐
☐

SLEEP

☐
☐
☐

GRATITUDE

NOTES

....
....
....
....
....
....
....

TIME	MEDICATION	DOSAGE	REACTIONS

DATE: ....

CHEMO DRUG: ....

DAY # ....   AFTER CHEMO # ....

TODAY I FEEL

EXERCISE

- [ ]
- [ ]
- [ ]

FOOD & DRINK

- [ ]
- [ ]
- [ ]

SLEE

- [ ]
- [ ]
- [ ]

GRATITUDE

NOTES

TIME	MEDICATION	DOSAGE	REACTIONS

DATE: ....

CHEMO DRUG: ....

DAY # .... AFTER CHEMO # ....

TODAY I FEEL

....

....

....

....

EXERCISE
☐
☐
☐

FOOD & DRINK
☐
☐
☐

SLEE
☐
☐
☐

GRATITUDE

NOTES

....

....

....

....

....

....

....

TIME	MEDICATION	DOSAGE	REACTIONS

DATE: ....

CHEMO DRUG: ....

DAY # .... AFTER CHEMO # ....

TODAY I FEEL

....
....
....
....

EXERCISE

☐
☐
☐

FOOD & DRINK

☐
☐
☐

SLEEP

☐
☐
☐

GRATITUDE

NOTES

....
....
....
....
....
....
....

TIME	MEDICATION	DOSAGE	REACTIONS

NOTES

NOTES

NOTES

NOTES

NOTES

NOTES

NOTES

NOTES

NOTES

Printed in Great Britain
by Amazon